50 Affirmations for People Who Choose to Take Medication for Depression and Anxiety

Saundra Jain, LPC, LMFT and
Rakesh Jain, MD

3 Cool Cats Publications

Publisher's Cataloging-in-Publication
(Provided by Quality Books, Inc.)

Jain, Saundra.
50 affirmations for people who choose to take medication for Depression and anxiety / Saundra Jain and Rakesh Jain. -- 1st ed.
p. cm.
LCCN 2001118666
ISBN 0-9713436-0-8

1. Depressed persons--Life skills guides. 2. Depression, Mental--Treatment. 3. Antidepressants--Side effects. 4. Affirmations. I. Title.

RC537.J35 2001 158.1
QBI01-701018

50 Affirmations for People Who Choose to Take Medication for Depression and Anxiety

 For information address: 3 Cool Cats Publications, 135 Oyster Creek Drive, Ste. G, Lake Jackson, Texas 77566.

ISBN 0-9713436-0-8
Manufactured in the United States of America

This book is dedicated to all the patients and families we have been privileged to know and work with.

ACKNOWLEDGEMENTS

This is our chance to say thank you to all the wonderful people who helped us bring this dream - our first book - to a reality.

Thanks in abundance to Lisa Gibson and Tonya Heard for their help and honest critiques in editing this work. We offer recognition and thanks to Sara and Mack Smith of U R Gems Group in Houston, Texas. Their book, *How to Self-Publish and Market Your Own Book*, plus our meetings provided us with direction and rekindled our interest in writing. Special thanks goes to Jean Zapalac of FotoGrafics in Lake Jackson, Texas for her help in instructing us on ways to tame and soothe our computer. To all our friends and colleagues who took time to read the manuscript and offer insightful, thoughtful comments, we offer our thanks and appreciation.

We express our deep and heartfelt gratitude to our parents. Their patience, encouragement, and never ending faith are the foundation for our many successes. Last, but definitely not least, we thank our son, Nick, for his support. His participation in forming **3 Cool Cats Publications** and his shared interest in writing makes this project a fun and rewarding experience.

Our spiritual growth, individually and as a couple, has definitely laid a strong foundation for this project to come to life. We are grateful and look forward to many promising and rewarding journeys.

INTRODUCTION

Today's world is fast paced and filled with opportunities and responsibilities. The topics of depression and anxiety are headline news and are frequently featured on talk shows like OPRAH. We now have a better awareness and understanding of these problems thanks to televised and written media. People are beginning to talk about these problems and seek help.

We work in the field of mental health. Saundra is a licensed professional counselor and a licensed marriage and family therapist. Rakesh is a psychiatrist. We are privileged to work with individuals and families who are struggling with depression and anxiety. A problem we deal with frequently is compliance with medication.

People are often resistant to the idea of medication due to perceived stigma, fear of ridicule, and shame. People quit taking their medication for many reasons such as side effects and lack of improvement. Others may stop taking their medication because they feel better but they are at risk of the symptoms returning.

We encounter these struggles on a daily basis. The patients' concerns and worries are varied and each deserves respect and consideration. We decided to write a book of affirmations for people dealing with the decision to take or continue taking medication for depression and anxiety. The book offers support and guidance when faced with this decision. This is an illness that affects entire family systems. Its impact far exceeds the boundaries of the family and reaches into the community, workplace, and social relationships.

This book offers positive affirmations to anyone confronted with the problem of depression and anxiety, especially when taking medication. We hope this book will serve as a source of strength for anyone who reads it.

Turn the page and begin your journey! It is filled with the power of choice and words promoting strength and health. Travel the pages with a sense of serenity and growth and know the journey is never ending.

Enjoy -

Saundra & Rakesh

Saundra & Rakesh Jain

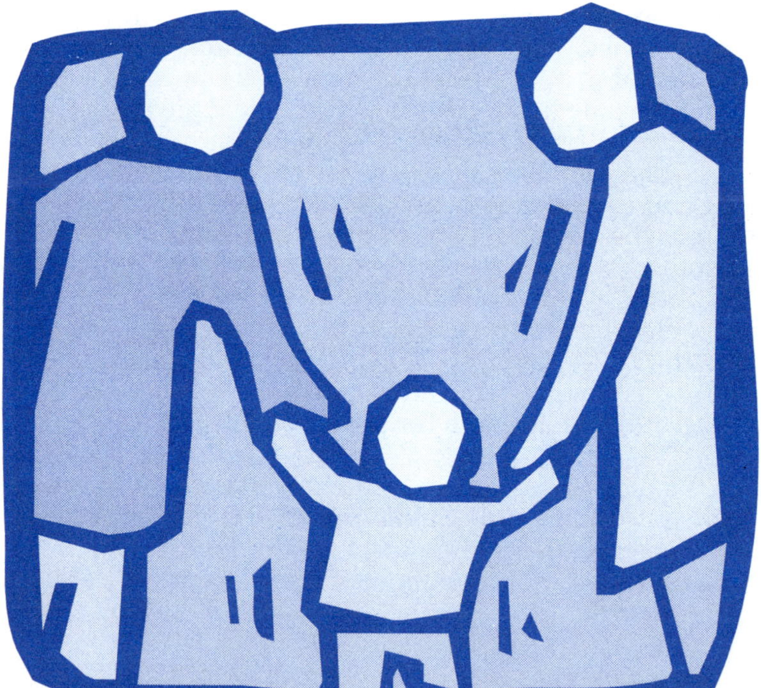

Medication assists me in dealing with depression and anxiety in a positive way. Medication enables me to deal with stress and day-to-day problems more effectively. Best of all, I am a better friend, spouse, and parent.

Saundra & Rakesh Jain

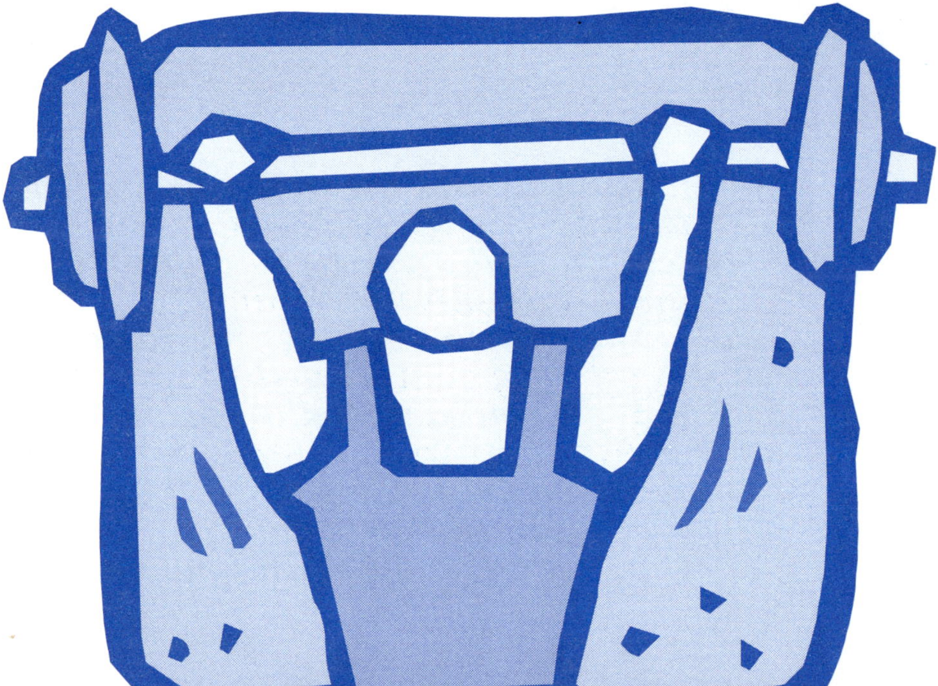

I promise to view taking medication as a sign of strength not weakness. It represents my commitment to health and a willingness to recognize a problem I can overcome.

Saundra & Rakesh Jain

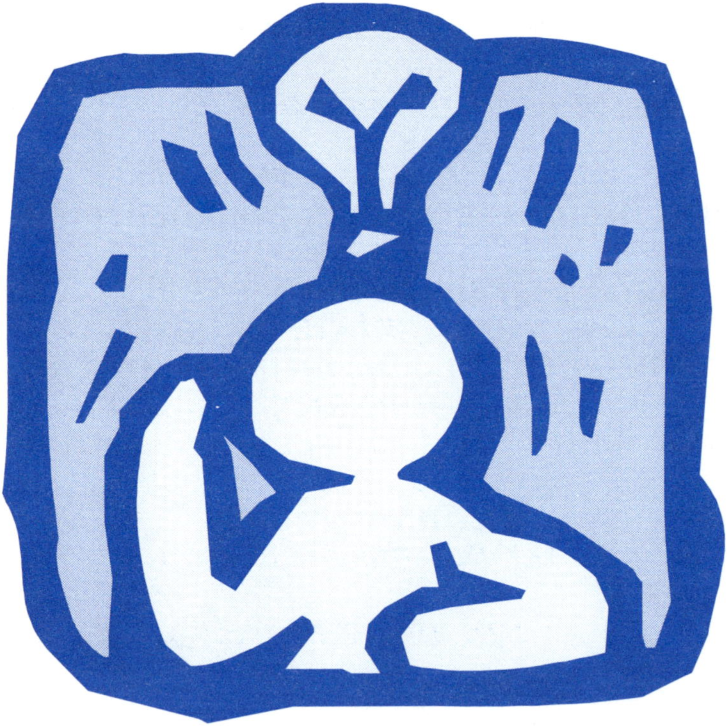

I recognize and accept the power of positive thought in my daily life. Positive thoughts counteract the negative thoughts associated with depression and anxiety. I will continuously train my mind to generate an abundance of positive thoughts. This I promise myself.

Saundra & Rakesh Jain

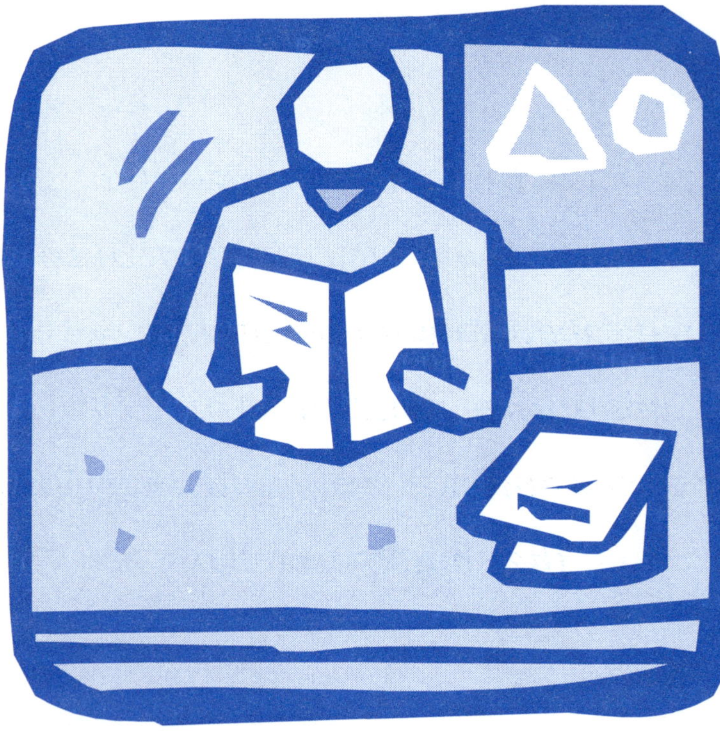

It is my choice to be on medication for depression and anxiety. I have educated myself about the illness of depression and anxiety and the available treatment options. I am empowered by the choices I make.

Saundra & Rakesh Jain

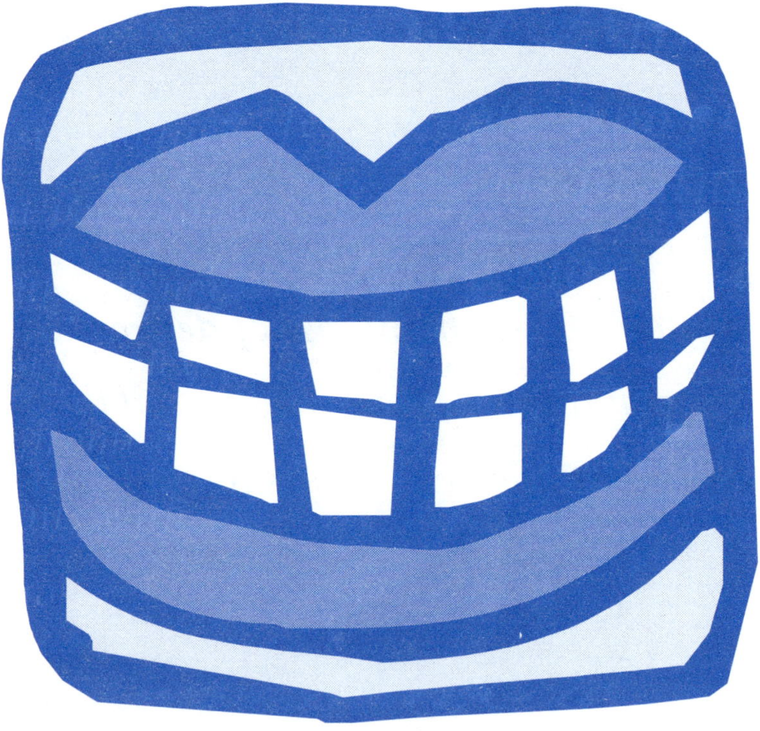

If others criticize my decision to take medication I will not take it personally. Their criticism will not hurt me nor steer me off course in my journey toward mental health. I promise to respond to their comments with tolerance and humor.

Saundra & Rakesh Jain

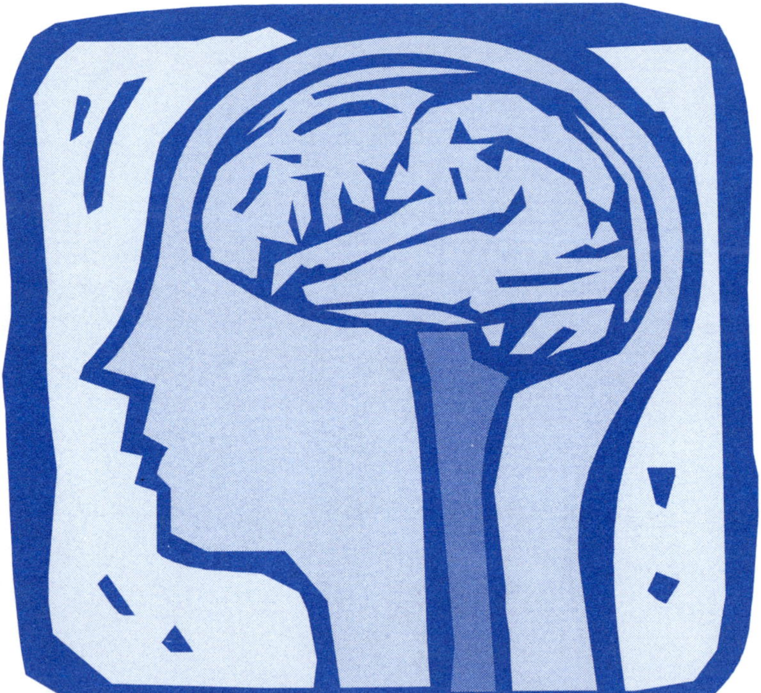

I believe people experience problems with depression and anxiety partly because of brain chemical dysregulation. Scientific data supports this belief. Medication helps me correct this chemical imbalance.

Saundra & Rakesh Jain

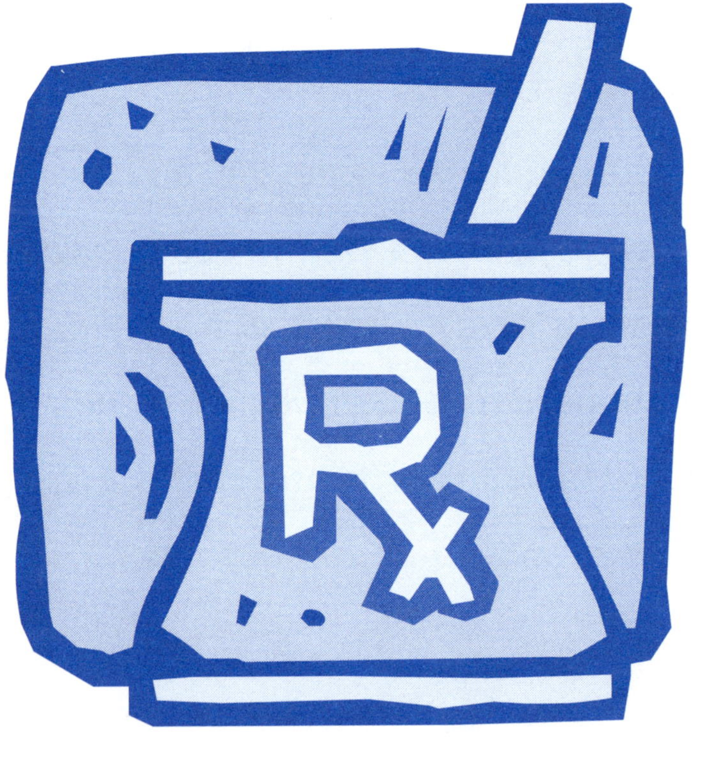

Some medications do not mix safely with other medications. Before I add any new medication, even over-the-counter medication, I will consult my physician.

Saundra & Rakesh Jain

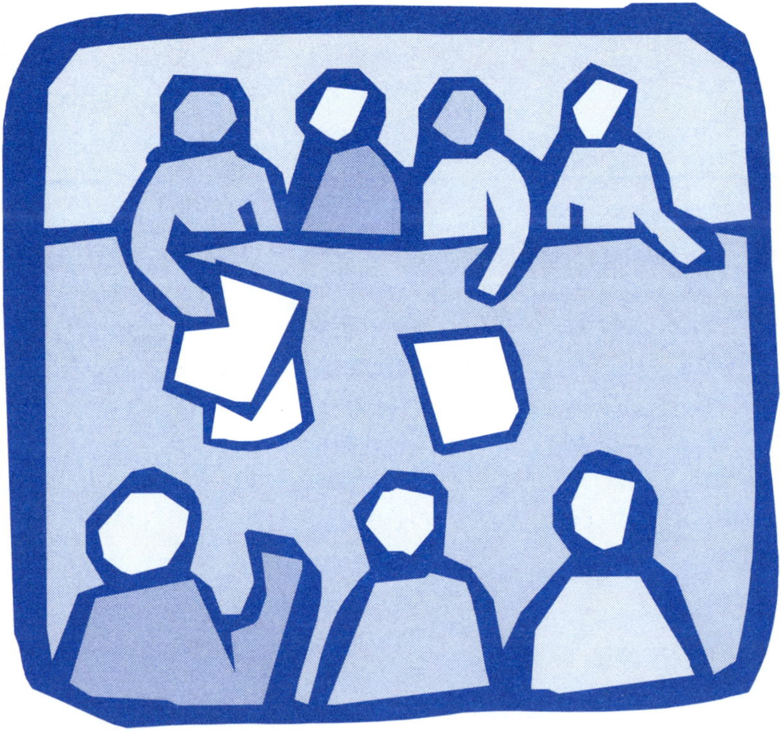

I am further empowered by joining support groups that are dedicated to serving the needs of people affected by depression and anxiety. In appropriate situations, I am an advocate for medication. Service to others furthers my healing.

Saundra & Rakesh Jain

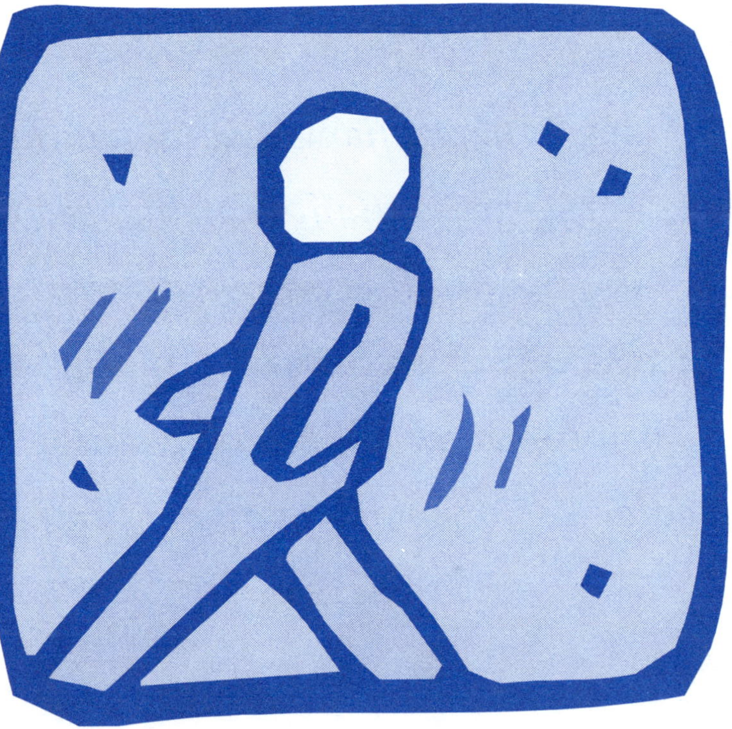

I gladly accept the benefits I receive from my medication. I will progress more quickly in therapy due to the reduction in depression and anxiety. I openly accept these benefits and continue to move forward with hope and anticipation.

Saundra & Rakesh Jain

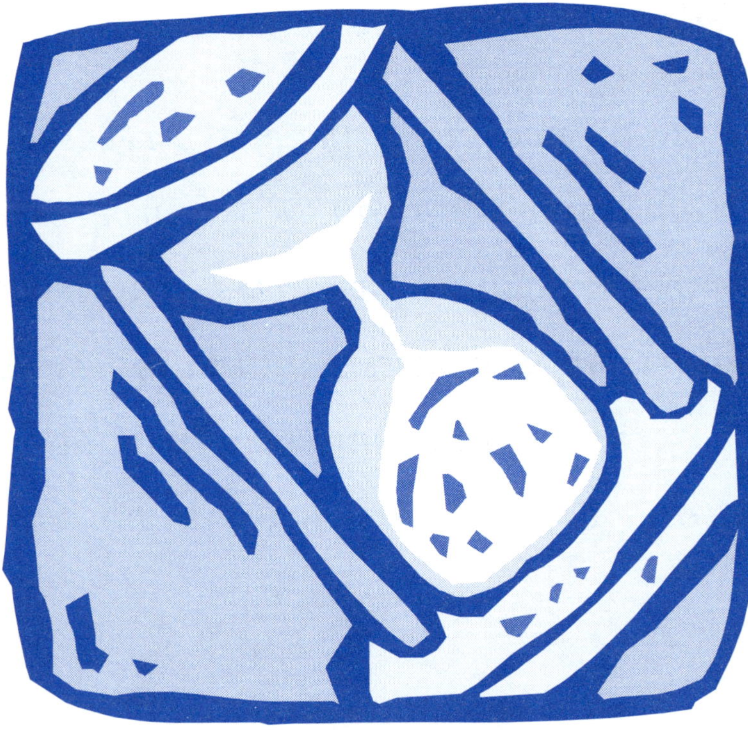

My patience is a virtue. It takes time to find the right medication and receive its full benefits.

Saundra & Rakesh Jain

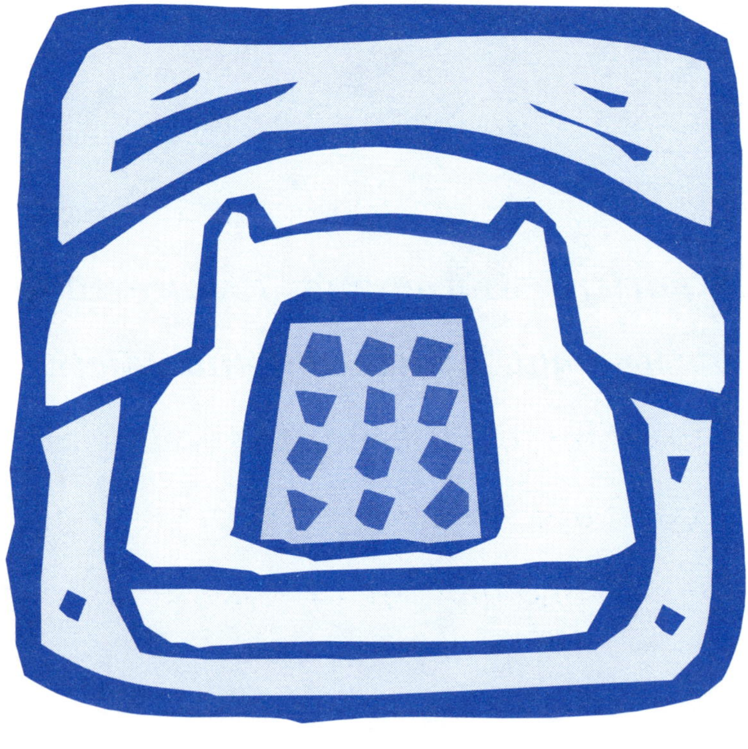

Taking medication for depression and anxiety is one way I choose to take care of myself. I will manage any thoughts of self-harm or suicide by immediately contacting my physician and therapist. I honor my life, cherish every moment, and relish each life-affirming breath.

Saundra & Rakesh Jain

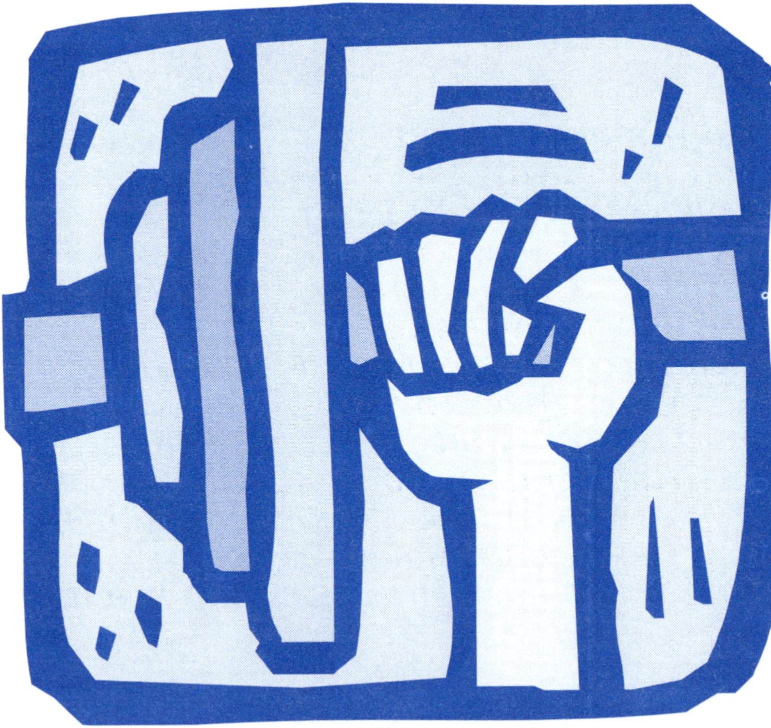

I honestly admit there are times I prefer not to take medication. My choice to take medication for depression and anxiety reflects my problem-solving attitude and wisdom. It is a sign of strength not weakness.

Saundra & Rakesh Jain

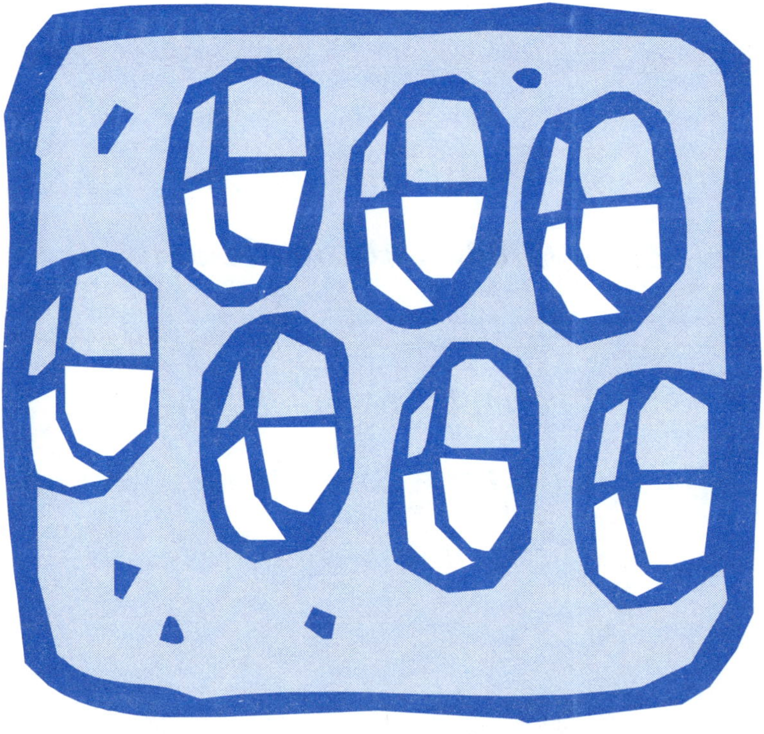

I accept the responsibilities associated with taking medication. I approach the duties of refilling prescriptions, calling my physician, and actively participating in all aspects of my care with a positive attitude. I envision and embrace the outcome of health and happiness.

Saundra & Rakesh Jain

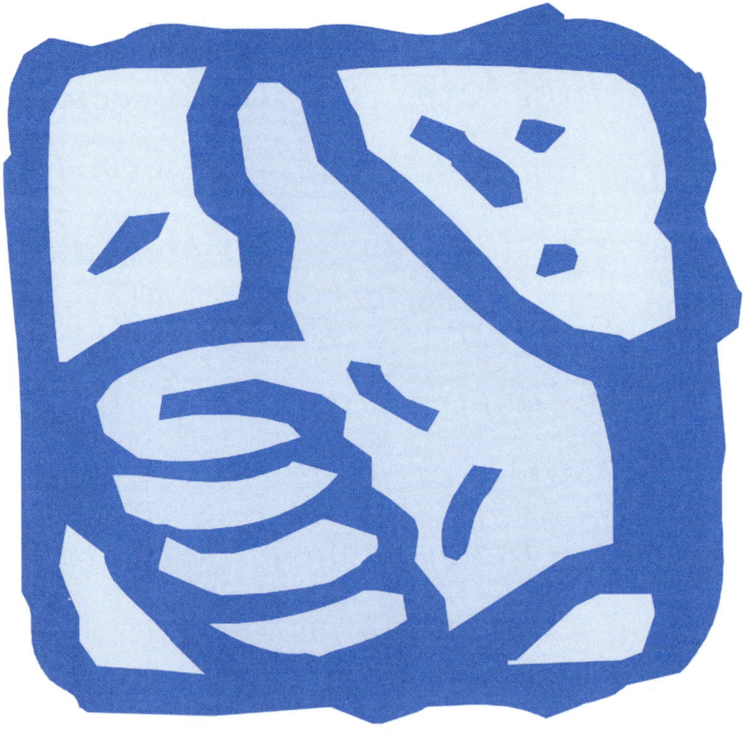

I believe in the power of my medication. This empowers me to change my life for the better.

Saundra & Rakesh Jain

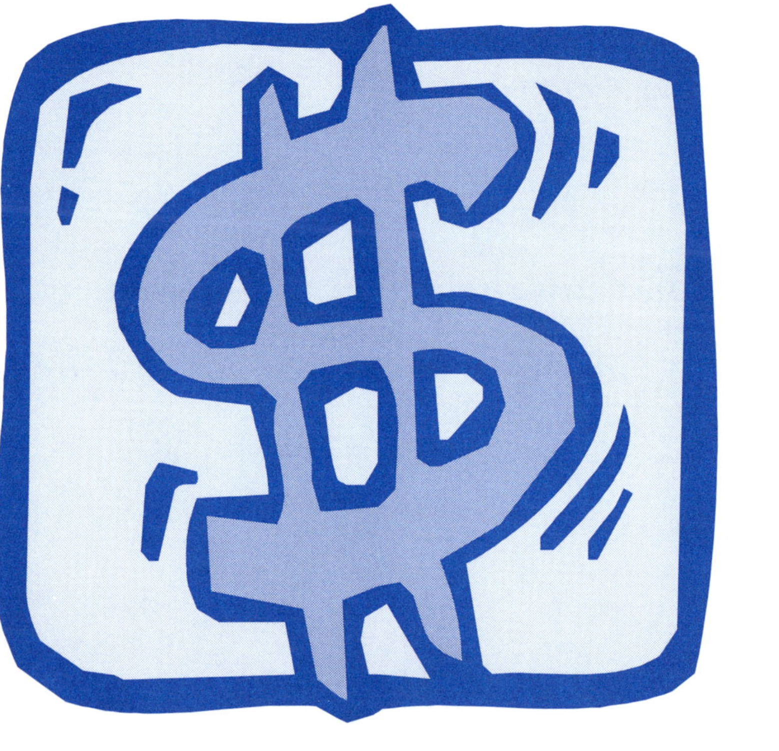

I may feel burdened by the financial stress of taking my medication. I will prioritize my needs and accomplish my goal of achieving good mental health. I am worth the investment.

Saundra & Rakesh Jain

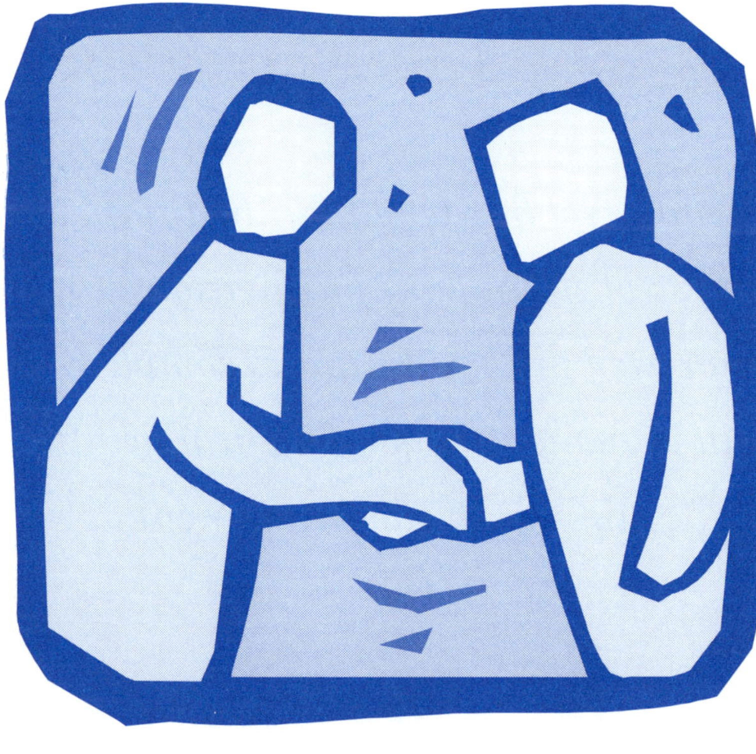

I am a positive person and believe in the power of partnership with my physician. This healthy partnership will allow us to use the medication to its fullest.

Saundra & Rakesh Jain

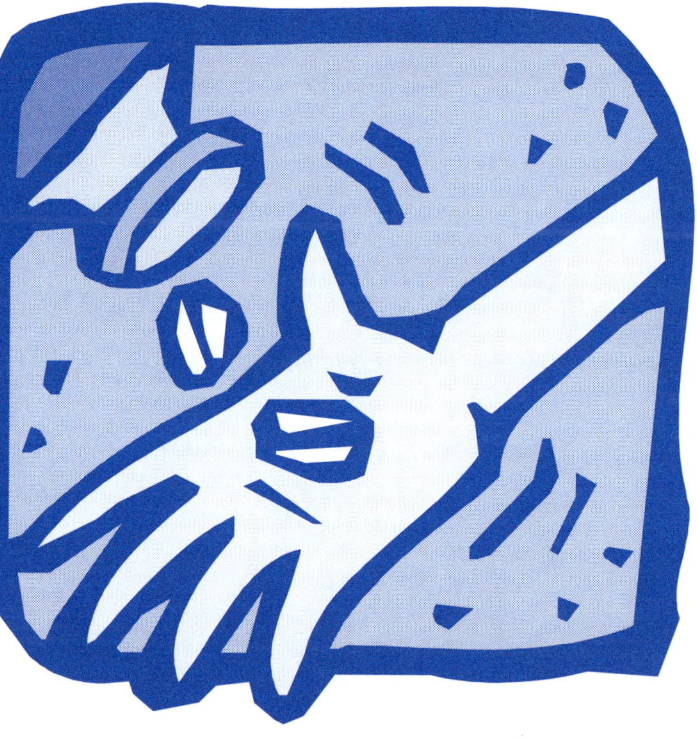

I respect all medications. I will take all medications responsibly.

Saundra & Rakesh Jain

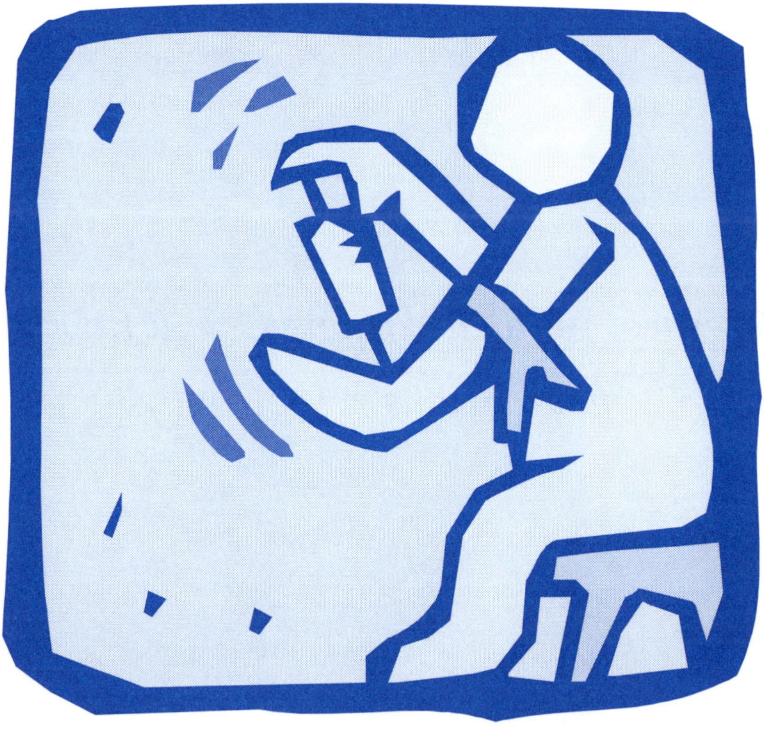

I am committed to leading a life free of addictions. I am aware all addictions are self-defeating behaviors. I will go forward with the help of my medication. I will not go backwards!

Saundra & Rakesh Jain

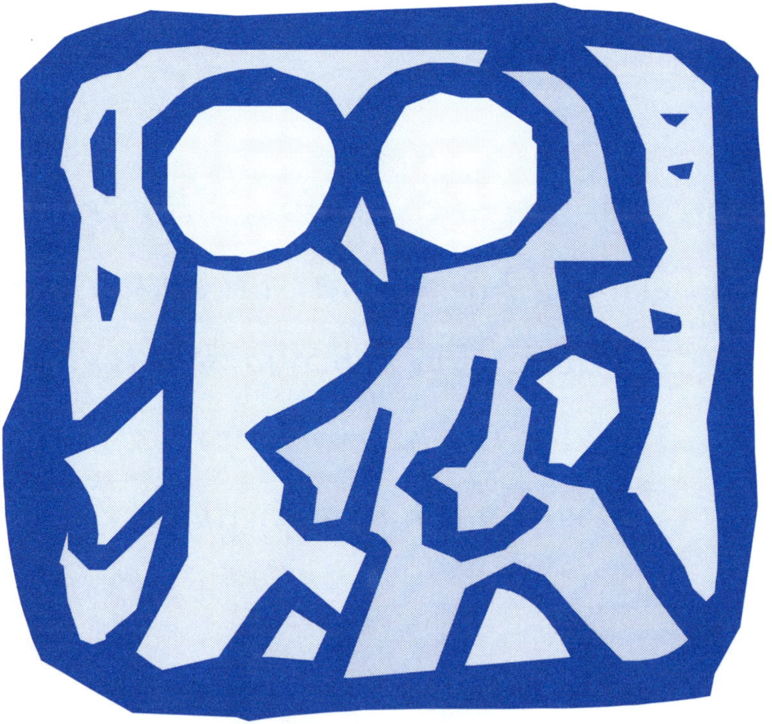

I am committed to friendships and socializing. I embrace the power to create and maintain friendships. Friendships are powerful aids in the fight against depression and anxiety. Utilizing this tool along with medication creates a strong defense. I feel empowered!

Saundra & Rakesh Jain

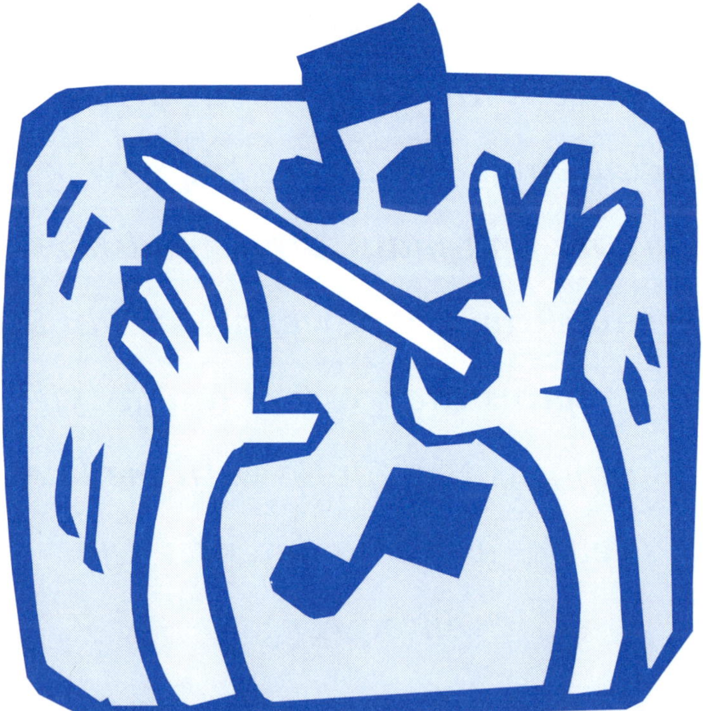

I will rely on each and every resource available to me: medication, exercise, good nutrition, therapy, spirituality, family, friends, work, faith... As these work in harmony, I can achieve anything!

Saundra & Rakesh Jain

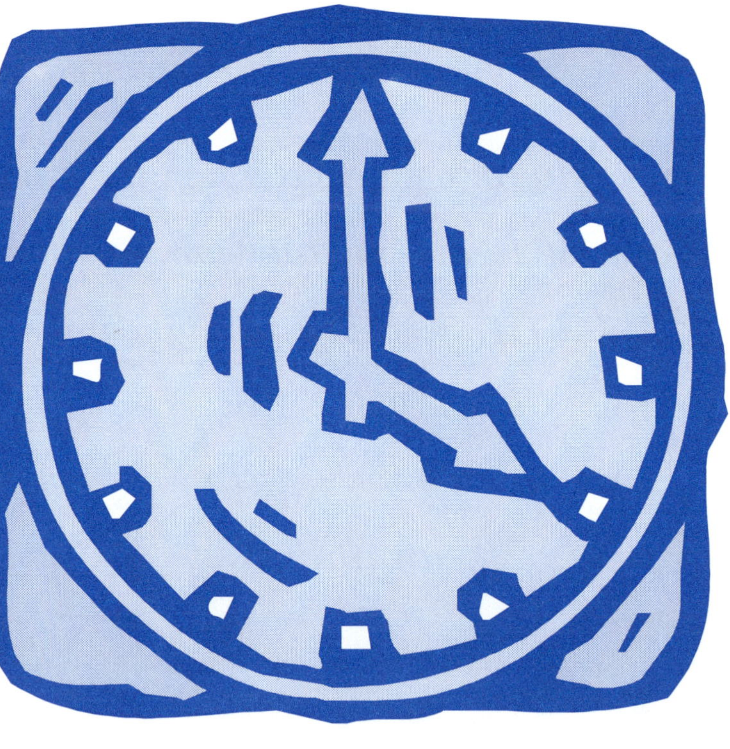

I accept the possibility of taking medication for an extended period of time if necessary. My knowledge has increased. I am a wiser person. If my physician recommends long-term use of a medication, I will remain flexible.

Saundra & Rakesh Jain

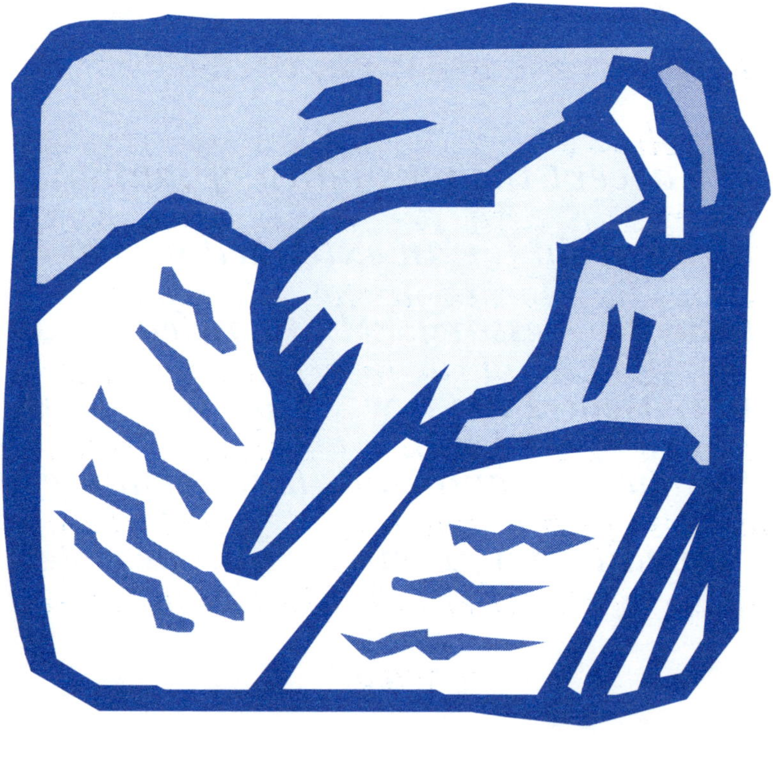

I am committed to education. I will teach my family and friends about mental health. I commit to helping others understand the role chemical imbalance plays in depression and anxiety. I will educate others about the benefits of medication. I will share my beliefs with others in a kind and gentle way.

Saundra & Rakesh Jain

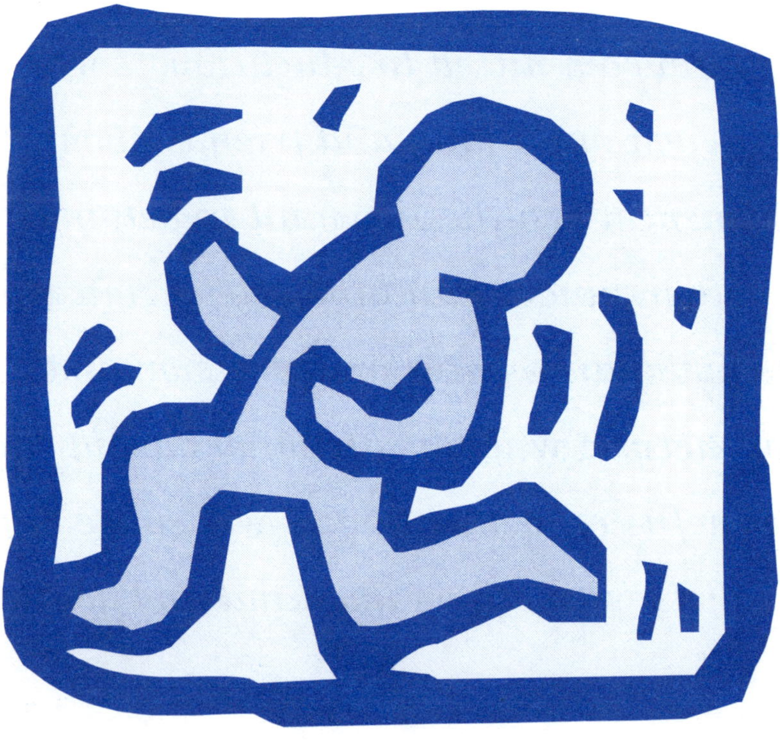

I commit to a physically active lifestyle. I will exercise daily. I will receive the full benefits of my medication as a result of this activity. So, I will commit myself to get moving!!

Saundra & Rakesh Jain

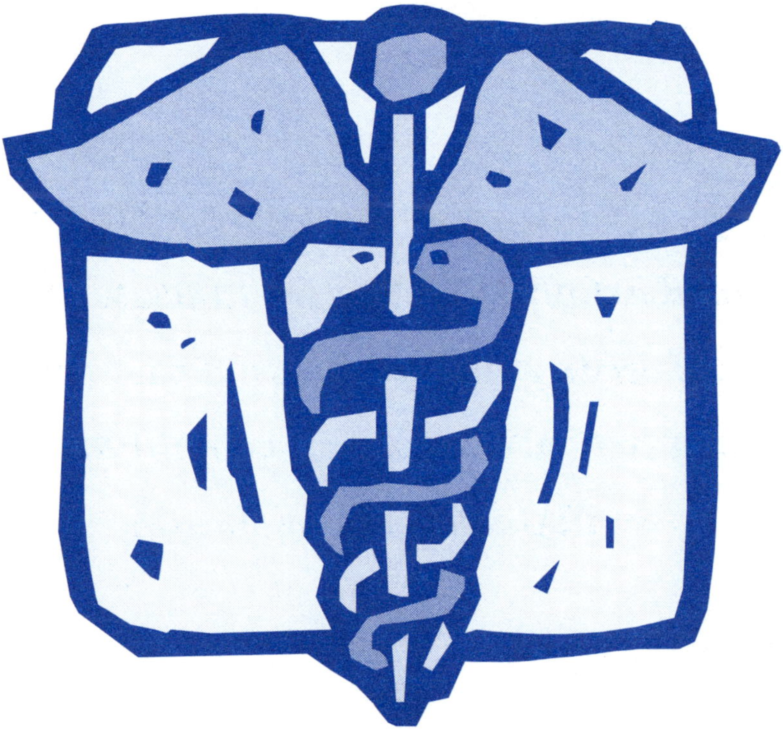

I believe depression and anxiety are medical illnesses, just like diabetes or any other physical illness. I view my medication the same way individuals with diabetes view insulin.

Saundra & Rakesh Jain

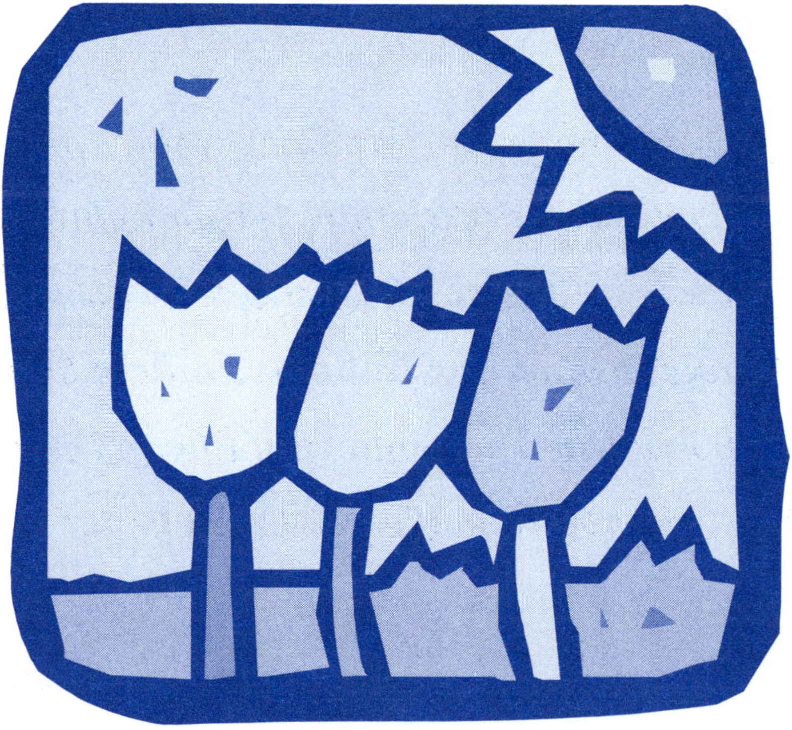

I will no longer criticize myself for needing medication. From today forward I accept this belief: "I choose to take medication so I can lead the best possible life. I honor my life and my ability to make good and sound decisions."

Saundra & Rakesh Jain

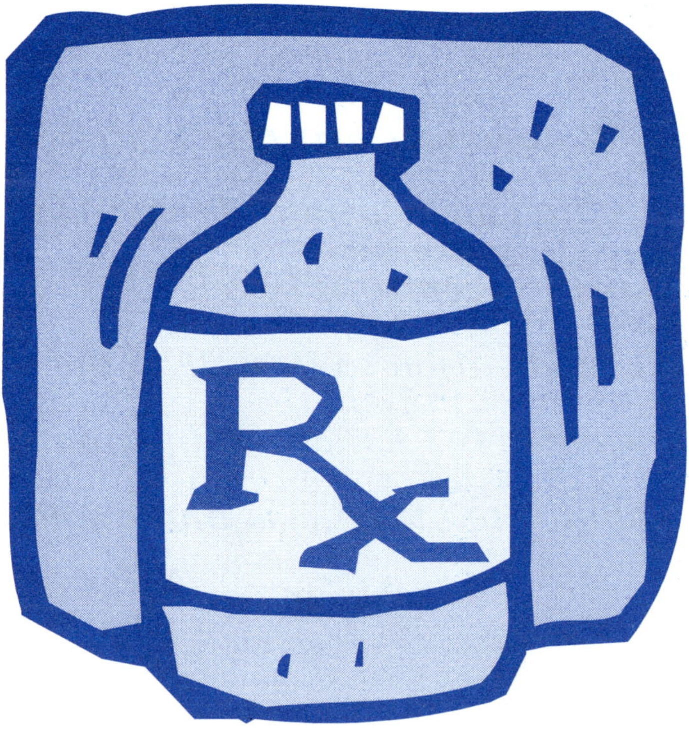

I promise to take my medication regularly and as prescribed. To not do so is to cheat myself. I am dedicated to taking great care of myself ---- forever!

Saundra & Rakesh Jain

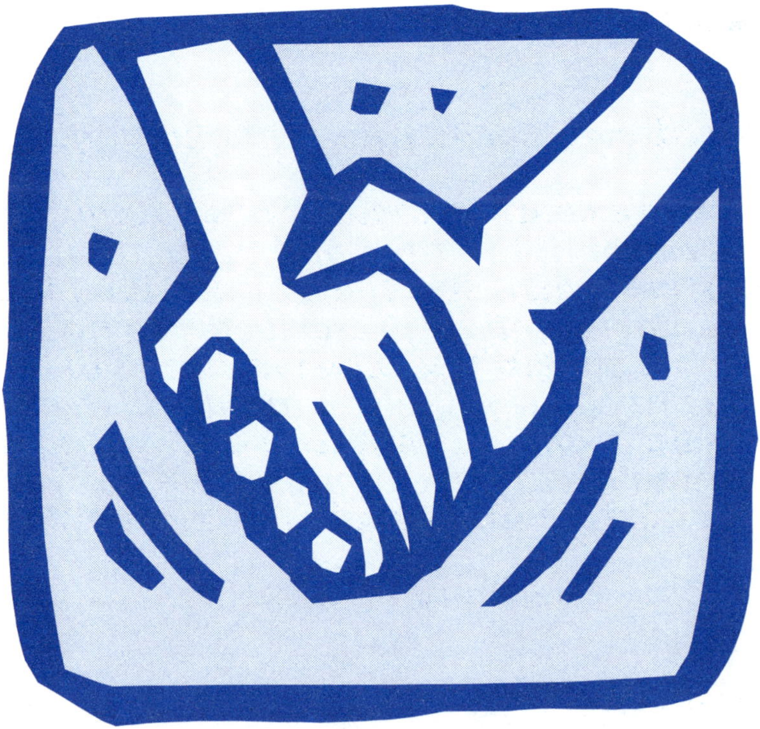

I will view medication in a kinder and more compassionate way. Anger, distrust, disrespect, and rejection play no role in my relationship with medication. I commit to developing a productive and beneficial relationship with my medication.

Saundra & Rakesh Jain

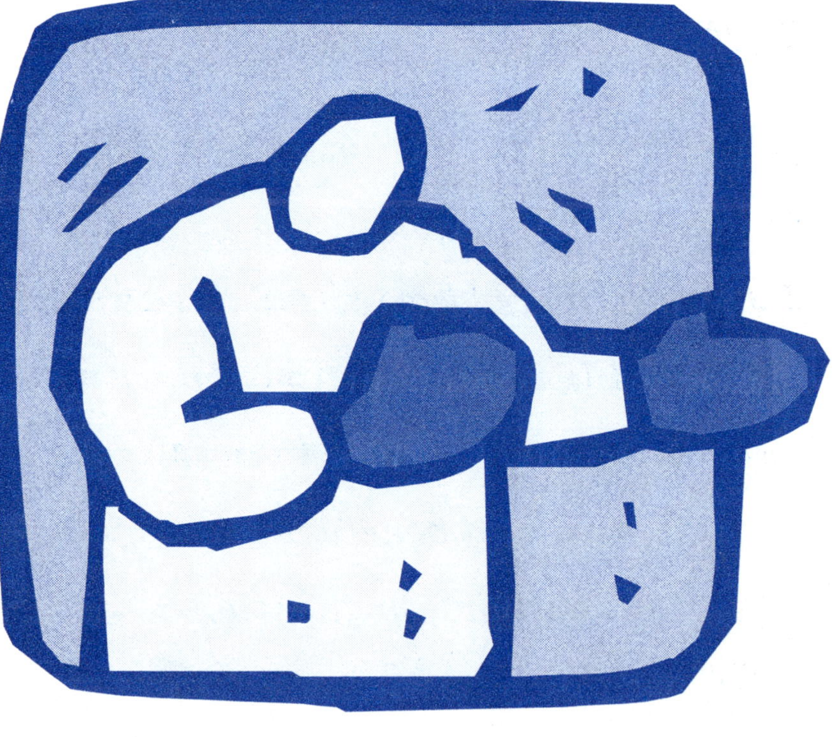

I am a fighter not a victim! Medication is one of the powerful weapons in my fight against depression and anxiety.

Saundra & Rakesh Jain

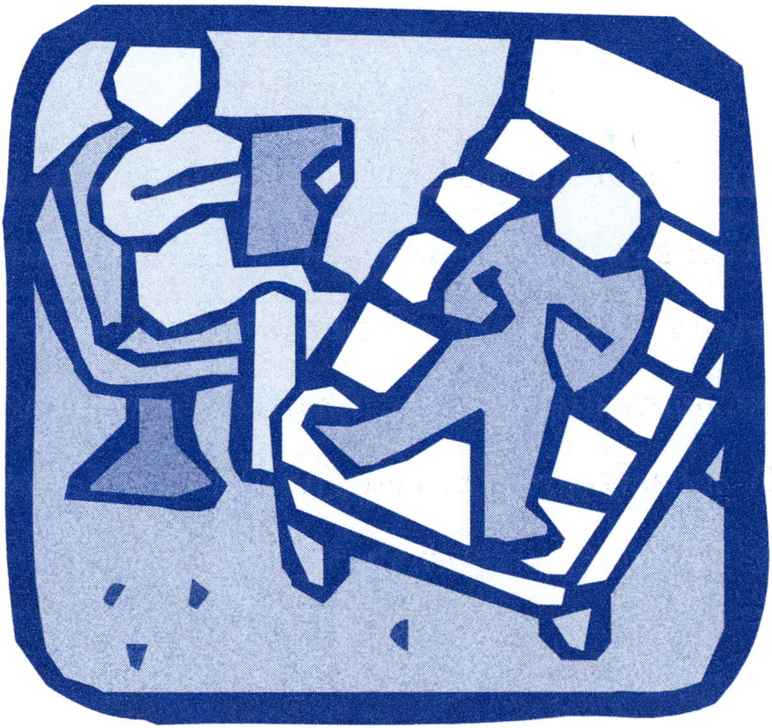

I am committed to search for a competent and compassionate physician and therapist. To truly benefit from medication and therapy I must feel listened to and cared for. I deserve only the best!

Saundra & Rakesh Jain

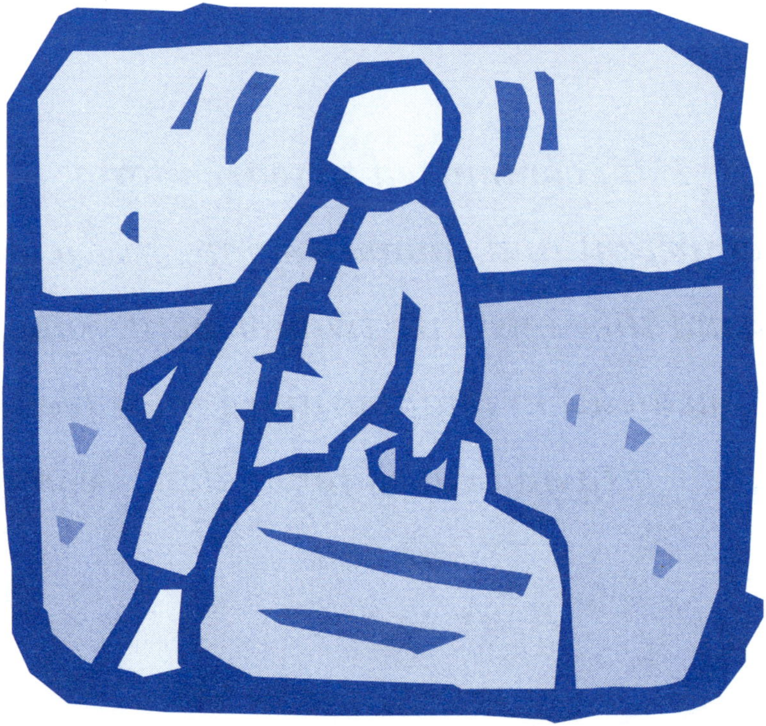

I choose to take care of my mental health and enlist the help of medication. Achieving the fullest potential is my goal. Medication supports my journey.

Saundra & Rakesh Jain

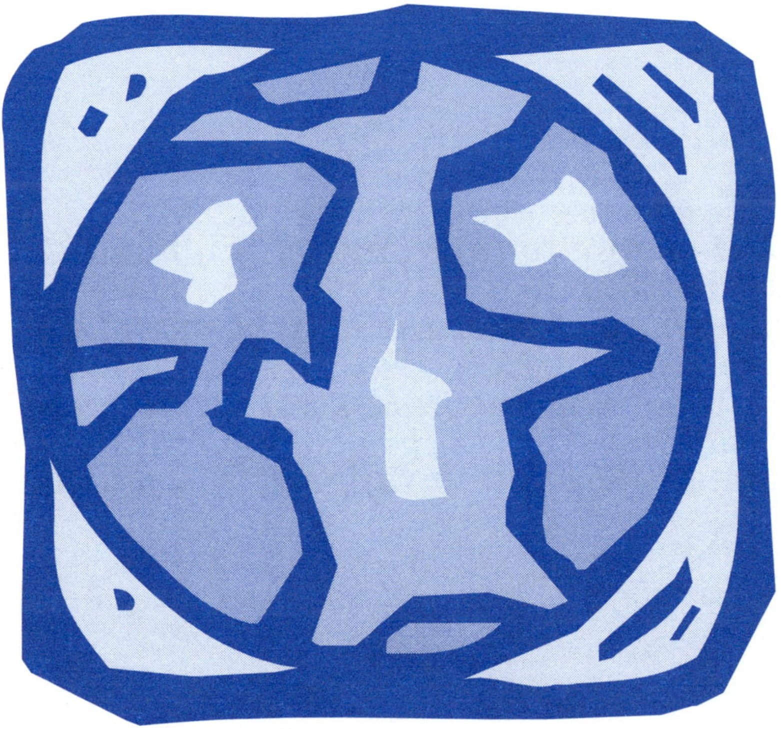

I know the world is not a perfect place. Even on medication my symptoms of depression and anxiety may resurface. I am not frightened by this possibility. I choose to maintain a calm watch over my moods and anxiety. I will keep my physician informed of any problems.

Saundra & Rakesh Jain

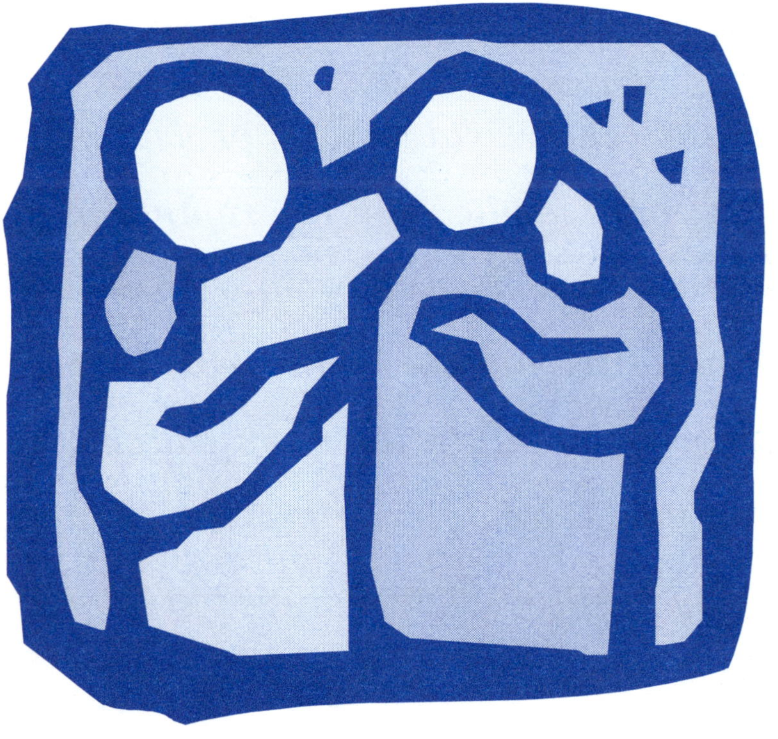

The relationship I have with my medication is like a friendship. Conflict plays a role in all friendships. I will learn to peacefully and respectfully resolve all conflicts. This friendship is one of joy, growth, and prosperity.

Saundra & Rakesh Jain

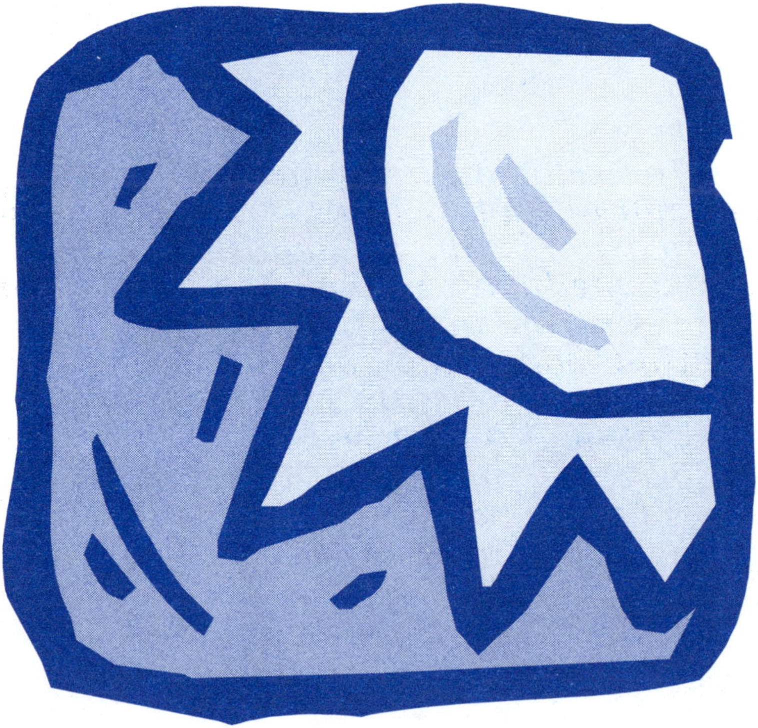

I do not accept feelings of shame because I take medication. I am nourishing my mind, body, and spirit in a journey toward health and wellness. Shame will play no part in this adventure.

Saundra & Rakesh Jain

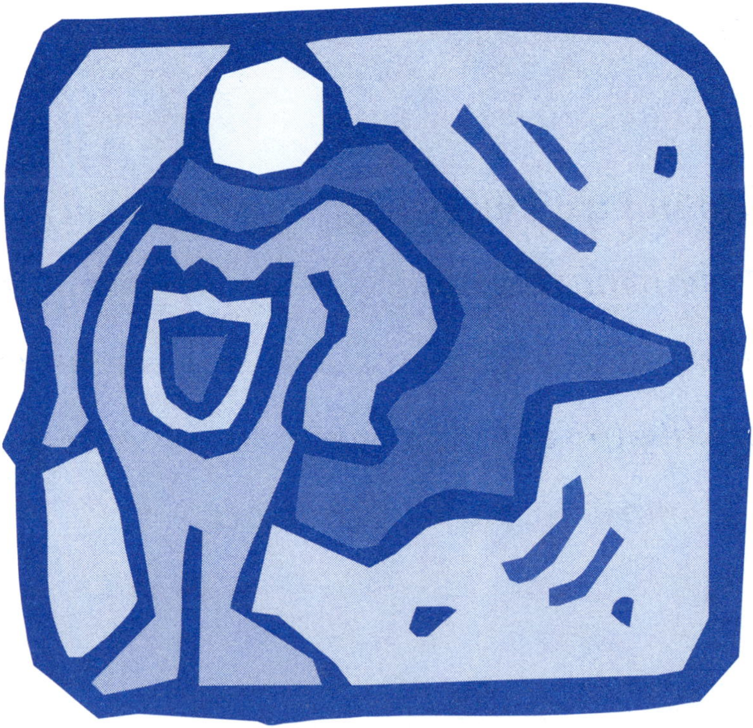

I am a role model for others dealing with the negative effects of depression and anxiety. I offer my guidance, support, and help to others interested in making positive changes.

Saundra & Rakesh Jain

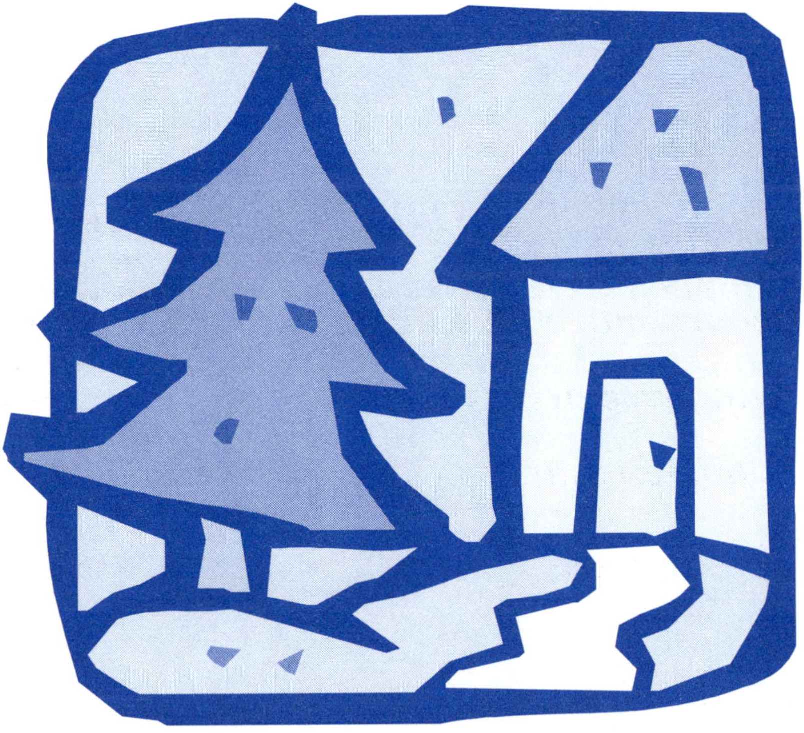

I will store my medication in a safe and secure place. No one, not even my pets, will have access to my medication. My home is safe for all those that enter.

Saundra & Rakesh Jain

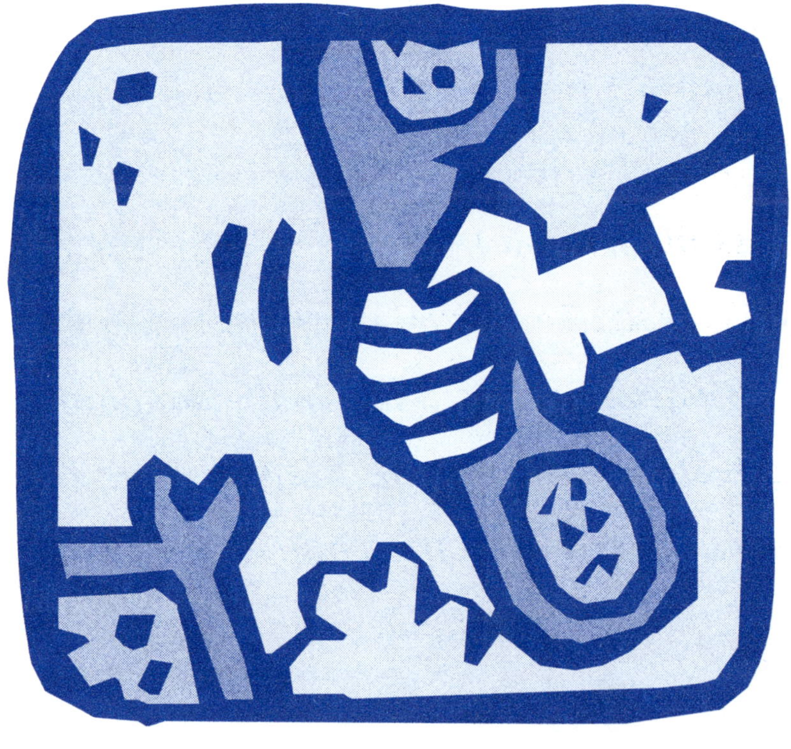

I commit to open communication with my physician. I am watchful for possible medication side effects. If they occur, I will report them to my physician immediately. Possible side effects might include sleep and weight changes, sexual life changes, nausea, headaches, etc.

Saundra & Rakesh Jain

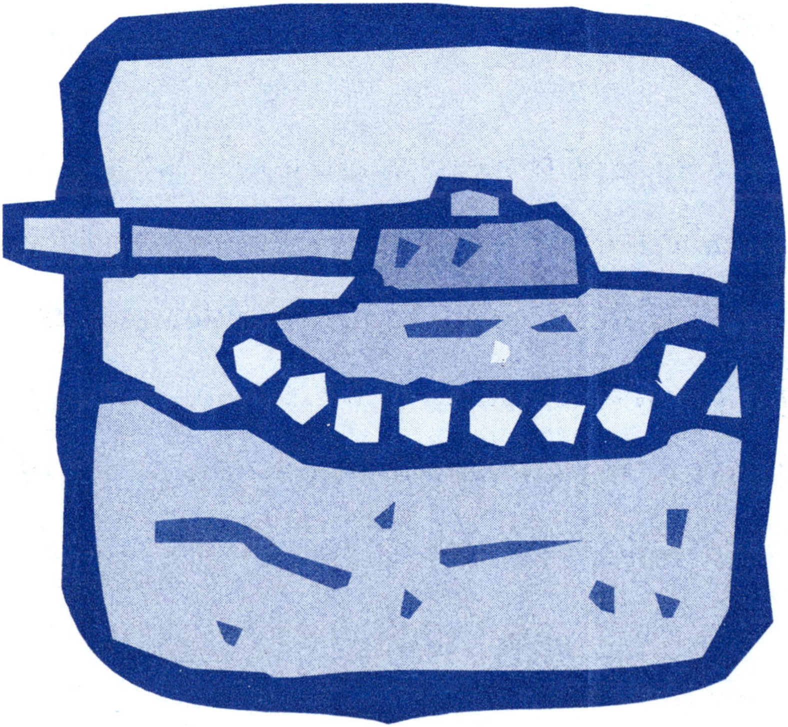

I recognize the destructive power of depression and anxiety. I am committed to doing all I can to harness this destructive force. Medication is one weapon I choose to use in my battle against depression and anxiety.

Saundra & Rakesh Jain

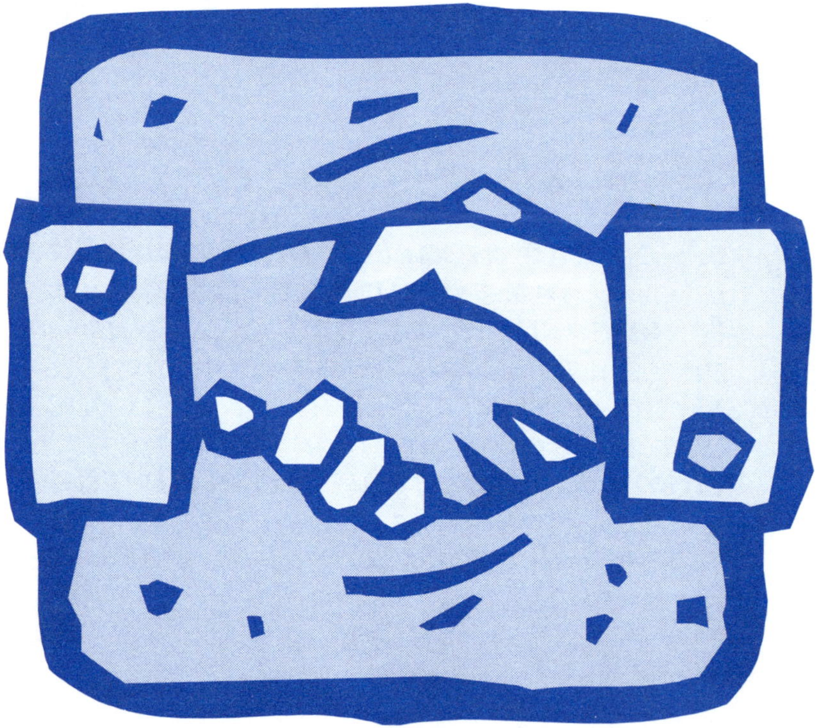

I know medication may cause side effects. I am committed to telling my physician about any problems I encounter. I benefit from the powerful partnership we share.

Saundra & Rakesh Jain

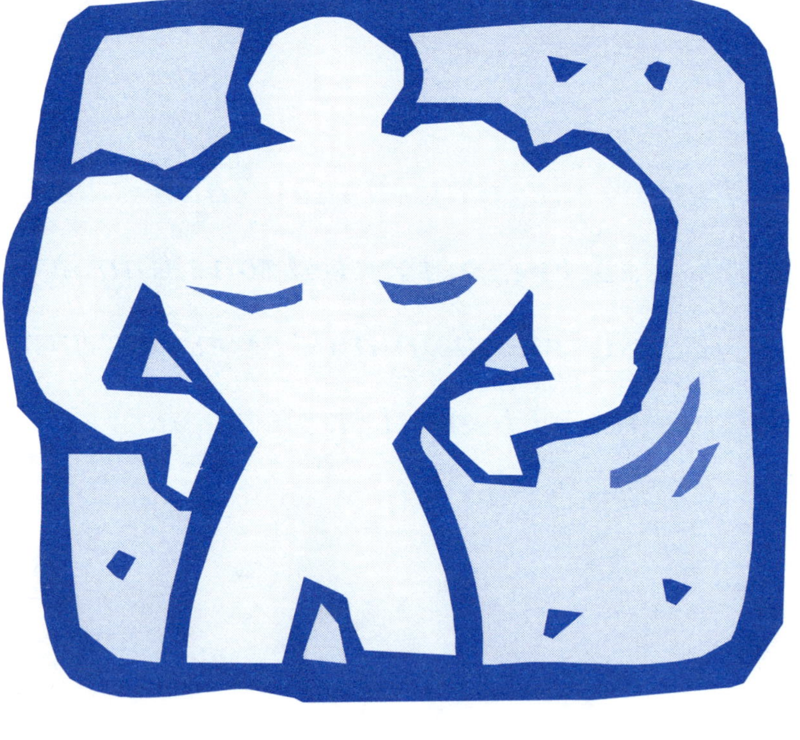

Medication makes me stronger in my ability to manage my depression and anxiety.

Saundra & Rakesh Jain

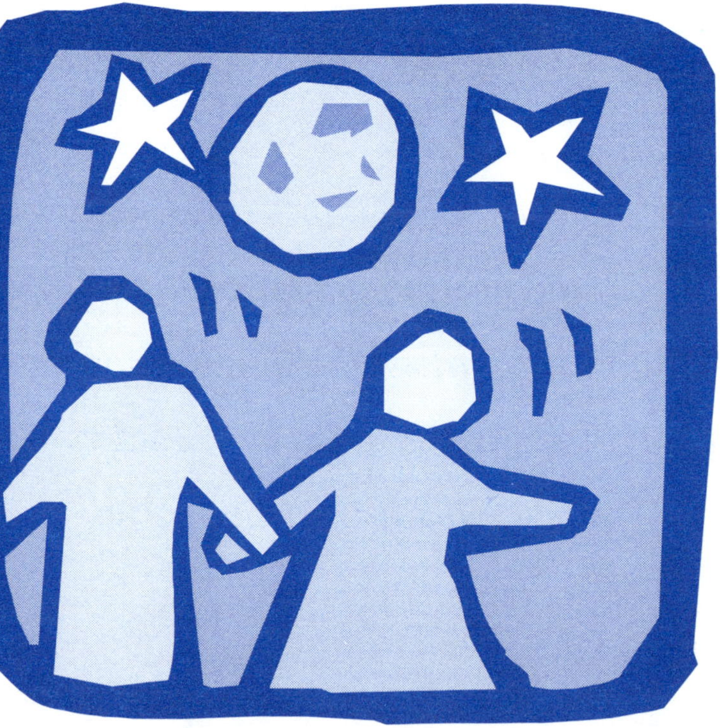

I commit to a balanced lifestyle. Medication helps me achieve this goal. I will also enlist the help of positive thoughts, positive actions, and positive relationships in my life.

Saundra & Rakesh Jain

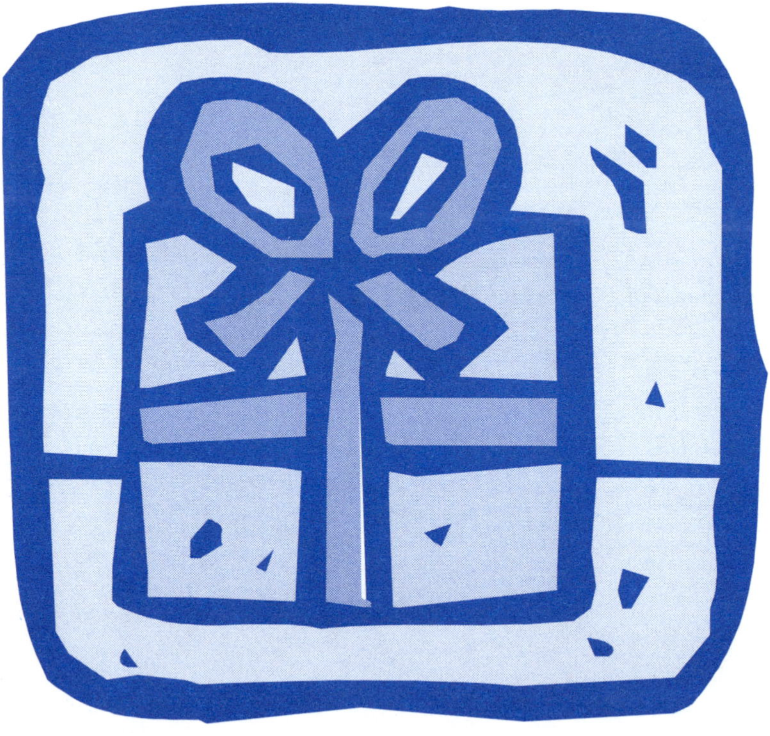

God's gifts are plentiful and abundant. Medication to control my depression and anxiety is one such gift. I freely accept the gift with gratitude and love.

Saundra & Rakesh Jain

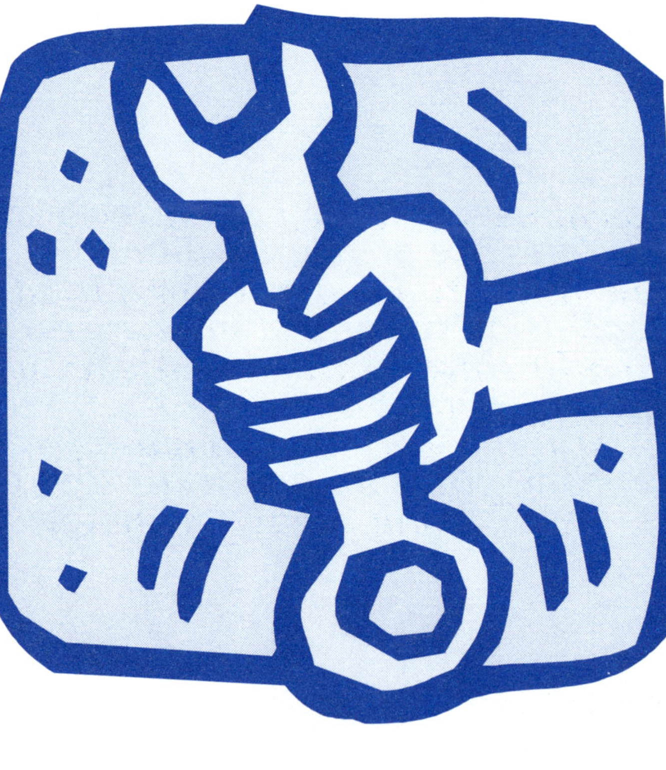

I recognize even the best of tools have their limitations. I am committed to doing all I can to ensure medications are successful for me. I will remain positive and strong in my journey.

Saundra & Rakesh Jain

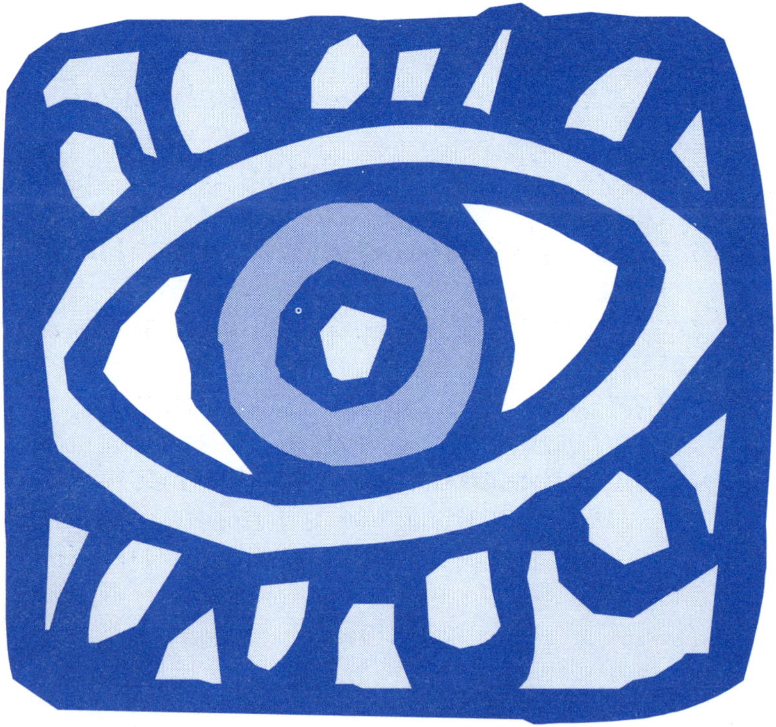

I promise to work cooperatively with my physician. If my physician and I agree to a trial of stopping my medication, I will proceed slowly and remain watchful for signs of depression and anxiety. I will follow my physician's directions. My goal is to protect myself in all endeavors.

Saundra & Rakesh Jain

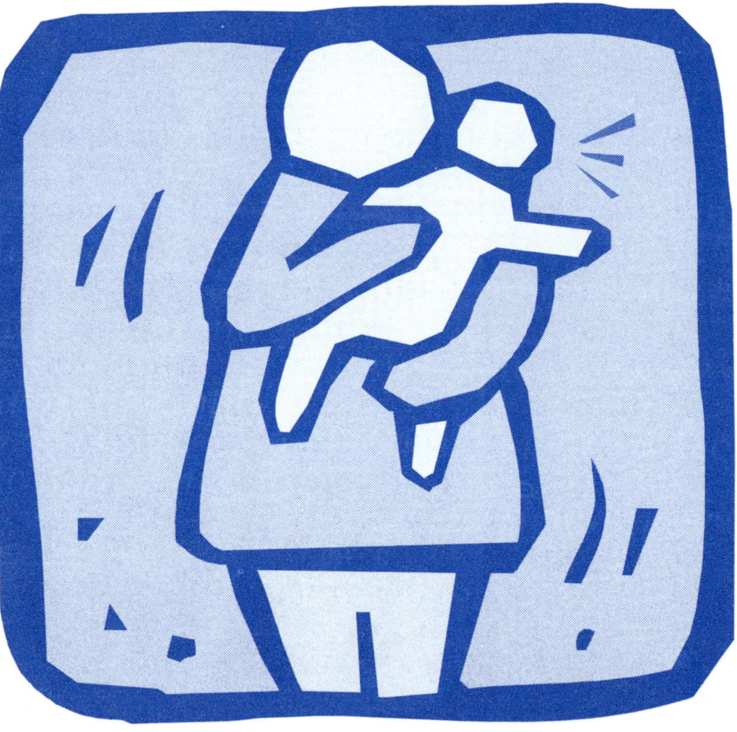

The decision to have a child demands thoughtful attention, especially while taking medication. I agree to discuss this option with my physician prior to making a decision. I am committed to the journey of health, growth, and prosperity.

Saundra & Rakesh Jain

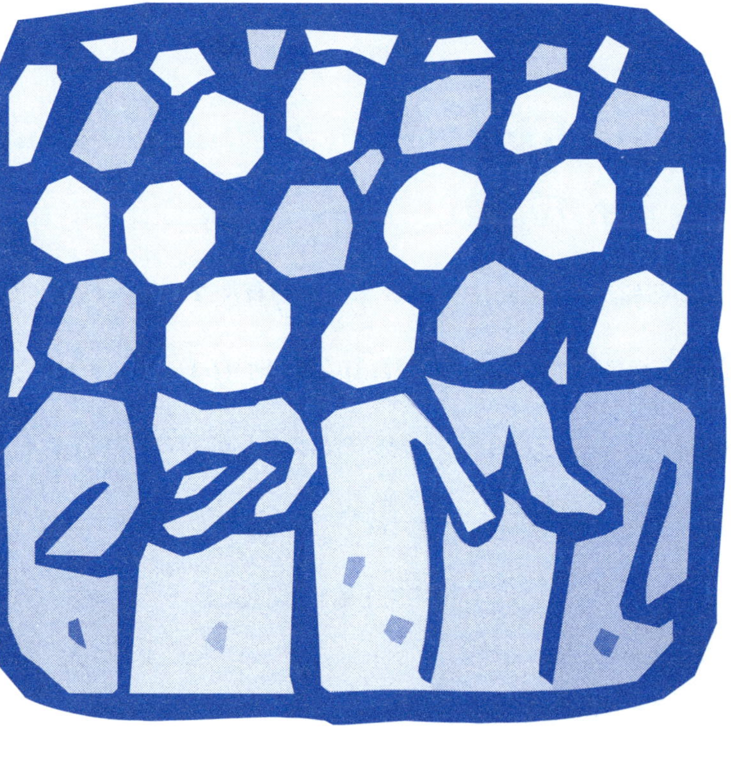

I acknowledge the benefits I receive from taking medication. Everyone in my life shares in the benefits.

Saundra & Rakesh Jain

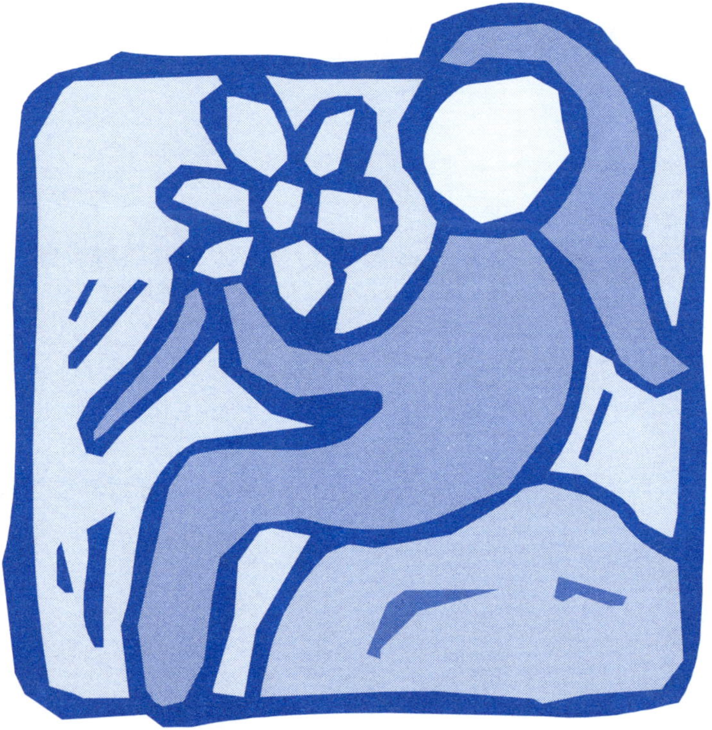

I am not defined by the medication I choose to take. To the contrary, wisdom, courage, and strength to make the right decisions to improve my life define me.

Saundra & Rakesh Jain

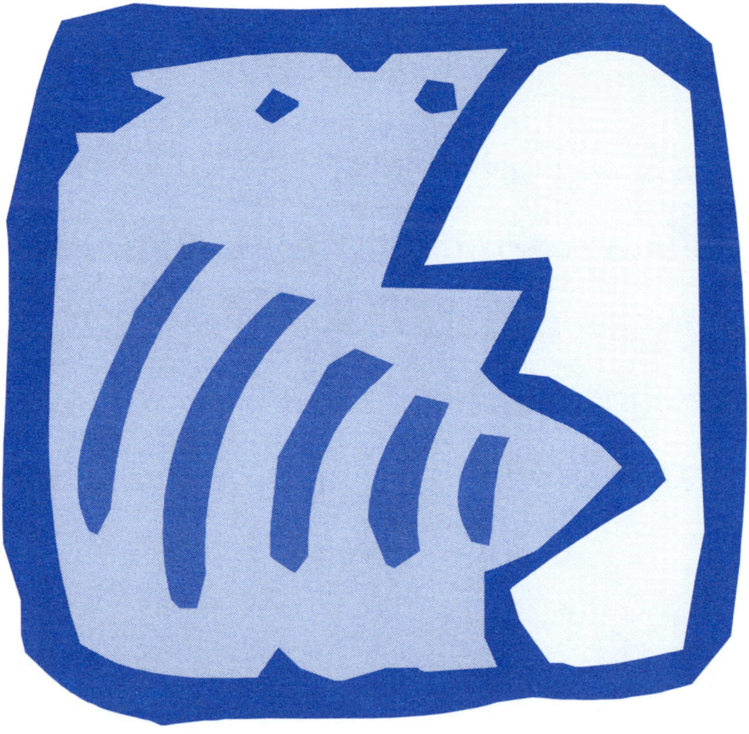

I will not stop taking my medication without consulting my physician. I am fully committed to my mental health and well being. I will talk to my physician before making any decisions about my medication.

Saundra & Rakesh Jain

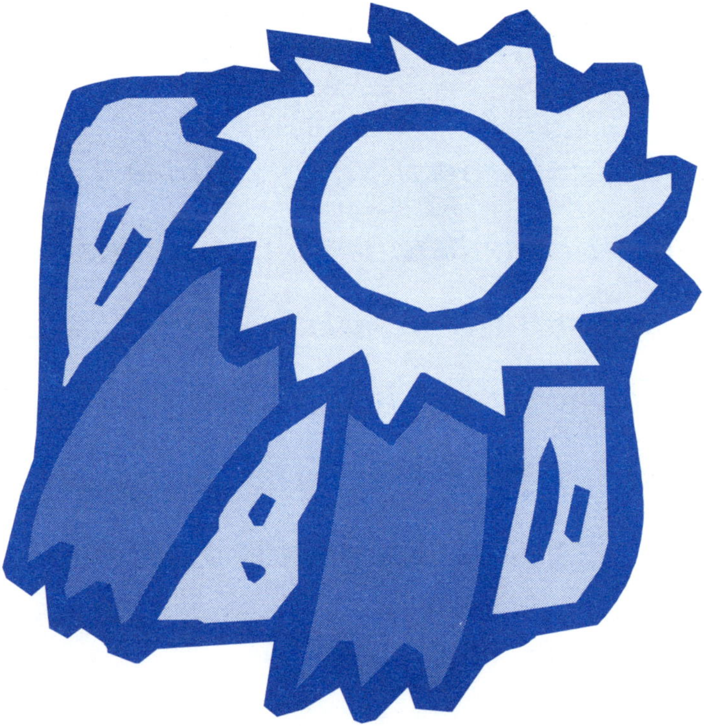

I do not choose to suffer from depression and anxiety. I am responsible for controlling the negative effect it has on my life and my family. My choice to take medication is one way I can win over depression and anxiety.

Saundra & Rakesh Jain

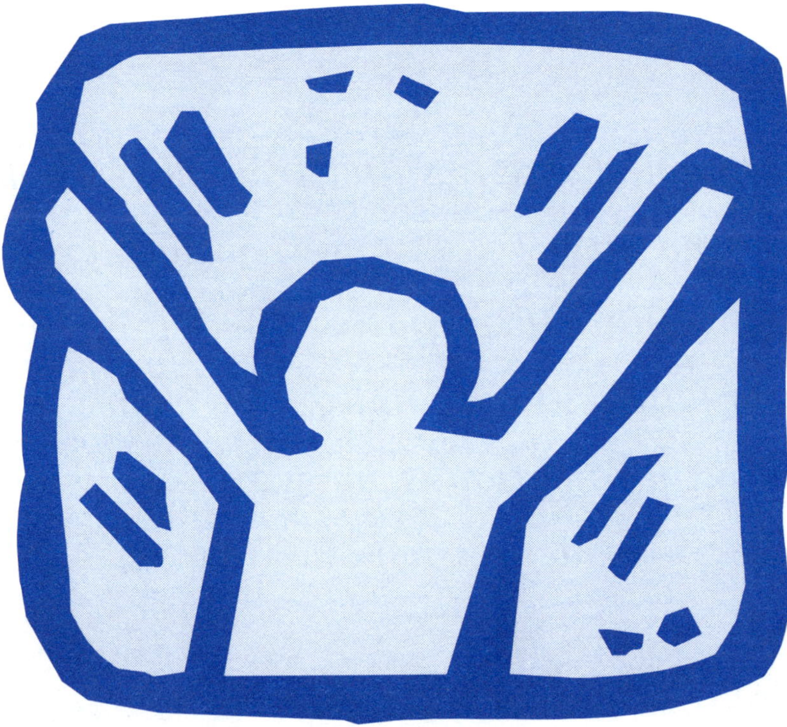

I commit to conquering depression and anxiety for the rest of my life. I will take advantage of all the tools available to me and continue to search for new ones. Medication is one of the tools available to me. I am blessed to have access to this powerful tool.

Saundra & Rakesh Jain

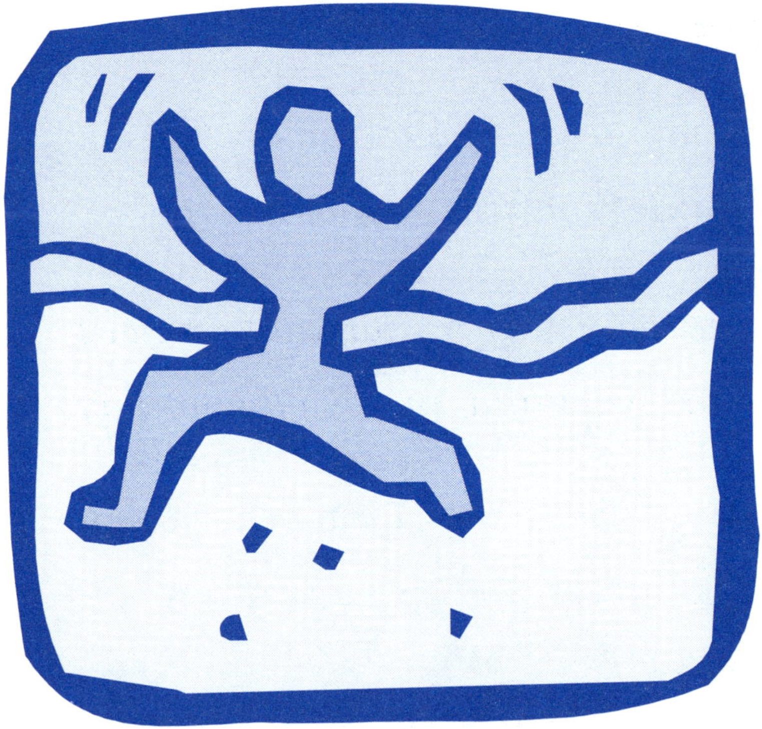

I have depression and anxiety.

Depression and anxiety do not have me!

ABOUT THE AUTHORS

Saundra Jain is a licensed professional counselor and a licensed marriage and family therapist. She graduated from the University of Houston at Clear Lake in Clear Lake City, Houston, Texas in 1984. She completed a Clinical Fellowship in Child and Adolescent Psychiatry at the University of Texas Medical Branch in Galveston, Texas in 1986. Saundra has worked in both inpatient and outpatient settings. Currently she is in private practice in Lake Jackson, Texas. She specializes in individual, family, and marital counseling.

Rakesh Jain is a psychiatrist with a Masters degree in Public Health (MPH). He received his degree from the University of Texas School of Public Health in 1987. He received advanced training in psychiatry from 1988 to 1993. Rakesh has received numerous awards and recognition for academic excellence, research experience, and teaching.

Saundra and Rakesh provide seminars, workshops, and community education on mental health issues including depression and anxiety. Their decision to pursue writing careers developed after people began requesting written information from their workshops and seminars. Their son, Nick Moore, is also interested in writing. Nick is in the seventh grade and is 13 years old.

3 Cool Cats Publications was formed as a result of Saundra, Rakesh, and Nick's shared interest in writing. And so began their writing careers. Saundra and Rakesh are currently working on a companion workbook to *50 Affirmations for People Who Choose to Take Medication for Depression and*

Saundra & Rakesh Jain

Anxiety. Nick is in the process of creating a children's book which teaches tolerance, respect, and good judgment.

The authors are available for workshops, seminars, and speaking engagements. Contact the authors at 979-480-9886 for more details.

3 Cool Cats Publications

Saundra Jain Rakesh Jain

Nick Moore

Saundra & Rakesh Jain

3 Cool Cats Publications

Quick Order Form

Telephone Orders: 979-480-9886 , Toll Free: 1-866-399-0329

Postal Orders: 3 Cool Cats Publications; 135 Oyster Creek Drive, Suite G,; Lake Jackson, Texas 77566

Website: www.3coolcats.net

Price of this book: $ 6.95

Please add $ 2.50 for shipping and handling for each book ordered. Texas residents please add 8.25% sales tax.

Payment:

- Check
- Type of Card (circle one) Visa, MasterCard, AMEX

Card Number ____

Name on Card: ____________________ Exp. Date___________